I0106086

Friendly Hedgehog Books

ISBN: 978-1-958622-15-5

Reach the authors at tlw@leadermakers.org

This Journal is the property of

_____

Please return to _____

_____

Email: _____

Phone: _____

Welcome

Welcome to *The Legacy Way: A Camino Training Journal*, designed to use alongside our book *The Legacy Way: Walking Into Purpose*. If you have not already obtained a copy of *The Legacy Way: Walking Into Purpose*, by Adam G. Fleming and Peter Jansen, it's highly recommended.

This journal is a place to record your thoughts, feelings, and data throughout several months. While it is designed for a Camino de Santiago pilgrimage, it can be used for walking on the Appalachian Trail, the Pacific Coast Trail, St. Olaf's Way in Norway, etc., or for making walking a regular practice at home. Feel free to use or ignore the quotes and questions. Write whatever is relevant to you each day!

You will find this book laid out in seven sections, as follows:

Section 1: Suggested Camino walking workouts, A list of hiking gear, and a 30-day Simulated Camino program for those who want to do a staycation Camino sabbatical experience.

Section 2: 90 Preparation Days. In this section, you'll have a question to consider for each of the 90 days of preparation. Note your workouts, other disciplines or habits, and if you have a *Legacy Way stamp,* give yourself a "passport stamp" for the Preparation stages just like the stamps pilgrims receive on the Camino de Santiago. *You'll also note that every 7th Preparation Day is marked as a Rest Day.*

Section 3: 3 Travel days. Travel to a hiking location is a time of separating from your home, family, work, etc. You're encouraged to reflect on how you're feeling as you drive, take a bus, train, airplane, ferry, cable car, or rickshaw as you voyage to your Camino experience location.

Section 4: 40 Camino days. Depending on which Camino or hiking trail you choose, you may not use them all. We've designed this section to accommodate pilgrims walking 34 days from St. Jean Pied-de-Pont and 6 extra to Finisterre and Muxia. *NOTE: skip to Day 40 when you*

ARRIVE at your final destination, whether Santiago de Compostela, Finisterre, Fatima, or wherever the hiking phase of your journey happens to end. If you have a shorter Camino feel free to do double journaling sometimes.

Section 5: 6 Camino Rest days. Turn to this section when you take a rest day during Camino.

Section 6: 3 Return Travel Days. A section to journal as you leave the Camino and return home.

Section 7: 30 Debrief days. Once you've completed preparation, a Camino, and about 3 weeks of debriefing, it's time to write out your LEGACY goal!

Appendix: Core Values Exercise

Buen Camino! From your friends,
Adam G. Fleming and Peter Jansen
Reach us at tlw@leadermakers.org

SECTION 1: WORKOUTS, GEAR, AND CAMINO SIMULATION SCHEDULE

PREPARING for your CAMINO: WALKING TRAINING PROGRAM

1. *At the beginning of each week, refer to this page to plan your walking into your schedule. Before going out for your walk, look at the journaling prompt to give you something to focus on as you walk.*

2. *After your walk(s), record your mileage/ kms in the journal and take 5-10 minutes to answer the journal questions.*

3. *You'll find a rest day once a week in the journal. (Day 7, 14, 21, and so on.) Here's a tip: I like to do my longer training walks on Saturday and Sunday, so I'll often use a midweek day like Monday or Tuesday for my recovery days. For example, if Monday is going to be your normal rest day, start this journal on a Tuesday, so that when the Rest Day comes, you're on a Monday. If you know your Camino start date, begin the journal as close to 90 days before that date as possible. There are six extra prep days in the journal in case you want to start a little earlier to time it up with your travel plans.*

4. *Review the program below and note that you'll gradually develop a need for twice as much time each week as you get closer to departure for your Camino. Begin thinking about what activities you're going to sacrifice so you don't get surprised by the intensity later.*

Training program in KILOMETERS

Week 1	5 days x 5 to 7 km	1 day x 8 km		38 km	7 hours
Week 2	5 days x 5 to 7 km	1 day x 10 km		40 km	7 hours
Week 3	4 days x 5 to 7 km	1 day x 10 km	1 day x 13 km	47 km	8 - 9 hours
Week 4	5 days x 7 km	1 day x 15 km		50 km	10 hours
Week 5	3 days x 5 km	2 days x 10 km	1 day x 16 km	51 km	10 hours
Week 6	3 days x 7 km	2 days x 10 km	1 day x 17 km	58 km	11 - 12 hours
Week 7	5 days x 7 to 8 km	1 day x 19 km		54 km	11 hours
Week 8	4 days x 7 to 8 km	1 day x 13 km	1 day x 20 km	61 km	12 hours
Week 9	4 days 8 to 10 km	1 day x 15 km	1 day x 19 km	66 km	14 hours
Week 10	4 days 7 to 8 km	1 day x 16 km	1 day x 20 km	64 km	13 hours
Week 11	4 days x 8 km	1 day x 15 km	1 day x 24 km	71 km	15 hours
Week 12	4 days x 8 km	2 days x 21 km		74 km	16 hours
Week 13	5 days x 7 to 8 km			35 km	7 hours

Training program in MILES

Week 1	5 days x 3 to 4 miles	1 day x 5 miles		20 miles	7 hours
Week 2	5 days x 3 to 4 miles	1 day x 6 miles		21 miles	7 hours
Week 3	4 days x 3 to 4 miles	1 day x 6 miles	1 day x 8 miles	26 miles	8 - 9 hours
Week 4	5 days x 4 miles	1 day x 9 miles		29 miles	10 hours
Week 5	3 days x 3 miles	2 days x 6 miles	1 day x 10 miles	31 miles	10 hours
Week 6	3 days x 4 miles	2 days x 6 miles	1 day x 11 miles	35 miles	11 - 12 hours
Week 7	5 days x 4 to 5 miles	1 day x 12 miles		32 miles	11 hours
Week 8	4 days x 4 to 5 miles	1 day x 8 miles	1 day x 12 miles	36 miles	12 hours
Week 9	4 days x 5 to 6 miles	1 day x 9 miles	1 day x 12 miles	41 miles	14 hours
Week 10	4 days x 4 to 5 miles	1 day x 10 miles	1 day x 12 miles	38 miles	13 hours
Week 11	4 days x 5 miles	1 day x 9 miles	1 day x 15 miles	44 miles	15 hours
Week 12	4 days x 5 miles	2 days x 13.1 miles		46.2 miles	16 hours
Week 13	5 days x 4 to 5 miles			20 miles	7 hours

PREPARING for your CAMINO: APPROPRIATE GEAR LIST

Procuring the proper gear for the Camino de Santiago is a major component of preparedness, roughly equal in importance to doing good physical training.

There are always variables, so ultimately you'll have to make some decisions on your own about things to leave at home or extras you feel are a must.

We'll break the list into two sections: clothing and pack/gear.

CLOTHING:

Shoes: the most important thing is to wear shoes that are broken in and know your own feet. I have narrow feet but a wide toe flair. I like to wear New Balance, although some might say they don't have a lot of padding, and they're not as sturdy as a hiking boot, they last forever and they give my toes room so that I don't develop blisters. If you train properly you should have an idea midway in your preparation whether the shoes you have will be good or not.

Lightweight flip-flops or Crocs for showers/evening time. Or sandals which can double as an alternative walking shoe in case your primary shoes cause a problem.

Socks: 4 pairs. We do NOT recommend cotton. Wool socks are far superior. Adam likes the Smartwool brand.

Pants: tactical pants, hiking pants, shorts – a lot of it depends on the season you're going to walk. Some people like to get the kind that have zip-off legs so you can convert to shorts. You can get by with two pairs, plus perhaps shorts to sleep in. In early spring or late fall, you may find yourself cold enough in lodgings to wear long pajama pants in bed. No cotton! If jeans get wet they're difficult to get dry. If hiking in warm weather take a swimsuit, invariably you'll want to jump in the water at some point because you'll feel like a kid!

Undergarments: 4 pairs of underpants. Ideally, stay away from cotton. However, I have used my normal cotton undershorts and it was fine. Check out blogs about hiking on the Camino if you're looking for advice on brassieres.

Tee Shirts: Three is adequate, four shirts are plenty. Again, no cotton. Use synthetics that dry quickly.

Long sleeves: depending on the season, you may want to bring a fleece, a light jacket, a windbreaker, or a raincoat. On Camino in February I found that I needed to purchase a fleece to stay warm at night, my raincoat over a tee shirt wasn't enough to keep me warm indoors.

Hat: I've used a baseball cap and wear it almost constantly. If you're walking in the summer and anticipate a lot of hot sun, avoid sunburns by using a broad-brimmed hat. You may not really like wearing hats, but take one anyway. A hat is better than a burn.

Gloves: in spring or fall, some lightweight gloves can be useful in the morning and evening.

PACK and HIKING GEAR:

Backpack: Even if you're going to transfer luggage with a bus every day, you'll want a day backpack for water, a sandwich, medicines, toilet paper, and other necessities. A fitted backpack with a belt in the 30- to 40-litre range is ideal for people who plan to carry everything with them.

Other bags: I take a light nylon string bag for general use, helpful for shopping, you may want a mesh bag to store dirty clothes apart from your clean ones, several gallon-sized plastic bags to keep clothes dry inside your backpack, and a shoulder bag, passport bag, or money belt.

Hiking poles: If you're listening to our podcast or watching us on social media you know that we can't recommend hiking poles enough. Several of our team thought they looked dorky until we tried them. They can "reduce compressive force on the knees by 25%." Anyone who has used them for a camino of over 150 miles will tell you they are a life-saver especially when going downhill. Think about it this way: if your pack is 15-20 lbs and adds roughly 10% to your body weight, putting extra pressure on your knees going downhill, the trekking pole will lessen the impact enough to more than neutralize the added weight of your pack. If you're going along with a group with The Legacy Way, poles are mandatory. That's how much we believe in them as a tool to avoid injury or unnecessary pain.

Poncho: There are special rain ponchos that extend to cover a backpack and it's critical to keep your pack dry if for no other reason than to keep your spare socks, underwear, and your sleeping bag dry.

Sleeping bag: unless you plan to stay in hotels every night you may need a sleeping bag. During the spring and fall it can get quite chilly, and even if you plan to stay in hotels, you might want a bag for extra warmth during spring and fall. Consider a silk liner and silk pillowcase to ward off bed bugs. Definitely take a pillowcase. Take an extra large plastic bag and put your sleeping case inside of it to double down on keeping it dry inside your pack.

Microfiber towel: gets you dry but dries out quickly. Also take a basic handkerchief or two, or a general-purpose rag, good for all kinds of things including wiping a bench or patio chair dry after a rain shower so you can sit down.

Small folding knife: only if checking your bags at airports! A small knife is useful for opening grocery store items and peeling fruit.

Tech kit: I take a MoKo Foldable Keyboard so I can type into a document or email on my phone, a battery pack that weighs almost a pound so I can recharge my phone in the wild (a small solar panel charger would work too) and a European adapter. Take your phone, though you'll want to think through and consider apps to temporarily delete while you're on the journey. A Garmin can be great for navigation when out of range for cell service in the forest.

Med kit: Prescription meds. Vaseline for your feet. A roll of toilet paper. Moleskin (Compeed), tape, and bandaids, for minor foot problems. Icy Hot for sore muscles. OTC meds like Pepto-Bismol tabs, ibuprofen, bandryl and Tums.

Toiletries: the usual, toothbrush and paste, soap, shampoo, comb, and deodorant. Don't forget nail clippers! I use disposable razors on Camino.

Paperwork: Passport and Camino 'credencial' plus cash, credit cards, guidebook (John Brierly's Guidebooks are great), and this journal with a couple of pens.

Water bottles: you may use a bladder with your pack that has a tube to drink from or you may want to use water bottles. I use the lightest ones I can get. You may want to start out the day with 2 or 3 liters. On the Camino, there are sometimes places to refill for free from a fountain with potable water.

From the hardware store or junk drawer: I like to take a couple of extra-long shoelaces. I've used them to fashion a makeshift clothesline, and of course, if a shoelace breaks you're covered. 6 or 8 clothespins to hang stuff on the line. Safety pins can come in handy as well, if you have wet socks and a sunny day you can pin them to your backpack and let the sun dry them as you walk.

Symbolic items: Many pilgrims take a small stone from home with them to put at a cross or some other mile marker to represent something they are leaving behind in their lives. You can also get a scallop seashell to carry on your bag (or buy a plastic one in Europe) to let people know you are a Camino pilgrim.

FOLLOWING PAGE: Thirty-Day Camino Experience Simulating Santarem, Portugal to Finisterre, Spain.
Walking days average 14.8 miles per day.

Activity	Depart	Arrive	KM	Miles
Walking day 1	Santarem	Amiais de Baixo	28	17.3
Walking day 2	Amiais de Baixo	Fatima	28.5	17.7
Walking day 3	Fatima	Caxarias	20	12.4
Walking day 4	Caxarias	Ansiao	26	16.1
Walking day 5	Ansiao	Rabacal	17.9	11
Walking day 6	Rabacal	Coimbra	29.2	18.1
Rest Day 1			0	0
Walking day 7	Coimbra	Mealhada	23.1	14.3
Walking day 8	Mealhada	Agueda	25.4	15.7
Walking day 9	Agueda	Albergaria a Velha	17	10.5
Walking day 10	Albergaria a Velha	Sao Joao	30.2	18.7
Walking day 11	Sao Joao	Porto	35.8	22.2
Rest day 2			0	0
Walking day 12	Porto	Vairao	23.5	14.6
Walking day 13	Viarao	Barcelos	30.9	19.2
Walking day 14	Barcelos	Lugar do Corgo	21.8	13.5
Walking day 15	Lugar do Corgo	Ponte de Lima	17.7	11
Walking day 16	Ponte De Lima	Rubiaes	19	11.8
Walking day 17	Rubiaes	Tui, Spain	18.4	11.4
Rest day 3			0	0
Walking day 18	Tui	Mos	19	11.8
Walking day 19	Mos	Pontevedra	28	17.3
Walking day 20	Pontevedra	Armenteira	21	13
Walking day 21	Armenteira	Vilanova de Arousa	23.6	14.6
Walking day 22	Vilanova de Arousa	Santiago	27.9	17.3
Rest Day 4			0	0
Walking day 23	Santiago	Negreira	21	13
Walking day 24	Negreira	Olveiroa	33	20.5
Walking day 25	Olveiroa	Cee	21	13
Walking day 26	Cee	Finisterre	14	9
Total			620.9	385

SECTION 2: PREPARATION DAYS

Preparation Day 1:
The journey of 1000 miles begins with a single step. – Confucius.
You've decided to make an incredible journey. How does it feel to get started?

TRAINING LOG: _____ miles or km _____ other training or disciplines

Preparation Day 2:

Let there be a vault ... God called the vault "sky" ... the second day.
-Genesis 1:6-7

Throughout a Camino journey you'll be outdoors a lot. Look up. Take time to notice the sky today. What do you notice about it that you haven't noticed for a while?

TRAINING LOG: _____ miles or km _____ other training

Preparation Day 3:

When the going gets tough, the tough get going. –Anonymous

Yes, it's an old cliché. Often the third day of a new routine or habit is the most difficult. You might be tempted... But don't skip today– get out and do something even if it's just for a few minutes. What was hard about getting out there today? Celebrate it, you're building momentum!

TRAINING LOG: _____ miles or km _____ other training

Preparation Day 4:

When the rate of change is higher than you're comfortable with, there could be stress. The key thing here is: You either mitigate, adapt, or suffer.
–Peter Jansen

Training is about mitigating pain. What other weak signals are you picking up from your body that indicate that you may want to mitigate more than just blisters? What else do you need to do to prepare?

TRAINING LOG: _____ miles or km _____ other training

Preparation Day 5:

I have nothing to prove, I have nothing to hide, and I have nothing to be afraid of. –Jason Potsander

What are you tempted to prove? What are you tempted to hide? What are you tempted to fear? How can you let go of these things today?

TRAINING LOG: _____ miles or km _____ other training

Preparation Day 6:

"The roots below the earth claim no rewards for making the branches fruitful."

— *Rabindranath Tagore*

As you walk or run today pay attention to the earth beneath your feet. Think about the legacy of the roots in the quote above. How can you be more like roots below the earth?

TRAINING LOG: _____ miles or km _____ other training

Preparation Day 7: REST DAY

"Where do we even start on the daily walk of restoration and awakening? We start where we are." ~ Anne Lamott

Take a rest day today and allow your body to recover. Write about how you can start where you are.

Begin considering core values. See the core values exercise at the
TRAINING LOG: _____ total miles completed in the last week.

Preparation Day 8:

"If you don't stick to your values when they're being tested, they're not values: they're hobbies." ~ Jon Stewart

Now that we're a week in and our preparation is in full swing, it's time to use the Core Values Exercise at the end of the journal and develop your top five.

TRAINING LOG: _____ miles or km _____ other training

Preparation Day 9:
"You have to have core values. What do you believe in? Do you believe in hard work? Do you believe in discipline? Do you believe in conditioning? Because those are the things I know that do work." ~ Tom Thibodeau

Maintaining your disciplines now is critical. In today's journaling exercise, list your #1 core value and discuss how you know when it is active in practical terms.

TRAINING LOG: _____ miles or km _____ other training

Preparation Day 10:

"The worst thing that could possibly happen as we get big and as we get a little more influence in the world is if we change our core values and start letting it slide, I can't do that. I'd rather quit." ~ Steve Jobs

In today's journaling exercise, list your #2 core value from your top five, and discuss how you know when it is active in practical terms.

TRAINING LOG: _____ miles or km _____ other training

Preparation Day 11:

"The minute you get away from fundamentals – whether it's proper technique, work ethic or mental preparation – the bottom can fall out of your game, your schoolwork, your job, whatever you're doing." ~ Michael Jordan

In today's journaling exercise, list your #3 core value from your top five, and discuss how you know when it is active in practical terms.

TRAINING LOG: _____ miles or km _____ other training

Preparation Day 12:

"The secret to achieving inner peace lies in understanding our inner core values – those things in our lives that are most important to us – and then seeing that they are reflected in the daily events of our lives." ~ Hyrum W. Smith

In today's journaling exercise, list your #4 core value from your top five, and discuss how you know when it is active in practical terms– as Smith says, how they are reflected in the daily events of our lives.

TRAINING LOG: _____ miles or km _____ other training

Preparation Day 13:

"I've learned my lesson hiring strictly on resume. At the end of the day, if they didn't match our core values, it was a disaster and I ended up losing other great people within the company - and that's time and money."
-Kendra Scott

In today's journaling exercise, list your #5 core value from your top five, and discuss how you know when it is active in practical terms.

TRAINING LOG: _____ miles or km _____ other training

Preparation Day 14: REST DAY

"It's very important that we re-learn the art of resting and relaxing. Not only does it help prevent the onset of many illnesses that develop through chronic tension and worrying; it allows us to clear our minds, focus, and find creative solutions to problems." -Thich Nhat Hanh

Allow your body to recover today. Rest by clearing you mind. As you focus, brainstorm ten or twelve potential solutions to a problem you're facing right now. Allow yourself to write down ridiculous ideas!

TRAINING LOG: _____ total miles completed in the last week.

Preparation Day 15:
"Change your practices without abandoning your core values." ~ James C. Collins

Now that you've had some rest and we're two weeks in, it may be time to increase your training. Your distance, speed or intensity... which means that your practices are changing. This means it's time to adapt, and that's going to be difficult at first. Journal about how you can do this without abandoning other core values.

TRAINING LOG: _____ miles or km _____ other training

Preparation Day 16:

"Winners embrace hard work. They love the discipline of it, the trade-off they're making to win. Losers, on the other hand, see it as punishment. And that's the difference." -Lou Holtz

What do you love about the discipline of the hard work you're doing today?

TRAINING LOG: _____ miles or km _____ other training

Preparation Day 17:

"Talent is cheaper than table salt. What separates the talented individual from the successful one is a lot of hard work." -Stephen King

Where are you most talented? What do you need to watch out for in terms of being tempted to lean on the talent?

TRAINING LOG: _____ miles or km _____ other training

Preparation Day 18:
"It's a conscious choice to challenge yourself." -Susie Young-Tatum
What conscious choices do you need to make today?
TRAINING LOG: _____ miles or km _____ other training

Preparation Day 19:
Expect the unexpected.
What have you noticed since you began this journal that you didn't
expect?
TRAINING LOG: _____ miles or km _____ other training

Preparation Day 20:

Plan some time in the next week for a long walk. A 'long walk' means something different to each person, but consider doubling the amount of miles or kilometers from a normal day. (If normal is 5 km, plan time to do 10 km.)

What will you need to give up to make that happen?

TRAINING LOG: _____ miles or km _____ other training

Preparation Day 21: REST DAY

As you take a break and allow your muscles to recover, stretch out a bit and feel your shoulders, back, legs ... where are you stronger than you were on day 1? (It may not be your body. It could be your mindset.)

TRAINING LOG: _____ total miles completed in the last week.

Preparation Day 22:

When we make progress and get better at something, it is inherently motivating. In order for people to make progress, they have to get feedback and information on how they're doing. -Daniel H. Pink

Where are you getting feedback on your progress? Who can you ask to encourage you?

TRAINING LOG: _____ miles or km _____ other training

Preparation Day 23:
If you do not conquer self, you will be conquered by self. -Napoleon Hill
What does it look like to conquer self today?
TRAINING LOG: _____ miles or km _____ other training

Preparation Day 24:
Quality is never an accident. It is always the result of intelligent effort.
-John Ruskin
What does it mean to do a quality job in your line of work? Where do you need to step up a notch?
    TRAINING LOG: _____ miles or km _____ other training

Preparation Day 25:

If you don't know where you are going, you might wind up someplace else. -Yogi Berra

As you train today consider the end that you have in mind. Imagine not knowing it for a while– if you didn't keep headed toward your chosen destination, where might you end up instead?

TRAINING LOG: _____ miles or km _____ other training

Preparation Day 26:

Notice that the stiffest tree is most easily cracked, while the bamboo or willow survives by bending with the wind. -Bruce Lee

In what ways do you need to become more flexible, more adaptable? How can you get there?

TRAINING LOG: _____ miles or km _____ other training

Preparation Day 27:

Life is full of beauty. Notice it. Notice the bumble bee, the small child, and the smiling faces. Smell the rain, and feel the wind. Live your life to the fullest potential, and fight for your dreams. -Ashley Smith

It's easy to get into a routine and then begin to not notice the smallest things. As you train today, notice something really small. Journal about the significance of that tiny thing you noticed.

TRAINING LOG: _____ miles or km _____ other training

Preparation Day 28: REST DAY

I have a vast 'bone pile' of stillborn or abandoned poems along with jottings and wisps from the great beyond that I tend to scan. Sometimes that leads somewhere, and sometimes the Muse is just on sabbatical.
-Maxine Kumin

It's a rest day, so you can try your hand at writing a jotting of a piece of a poem. Or, you can skip your journaling today if you want. Even full-time writers don't write every day.

TRAINING LOG: _____ total miles completed in the last week.

Preparation Day 29:

No matter what happens in life, be good to people. Being good to people is a wonderful legacy to leave behind. -Taylor Swift

Where is one area of your life where you can choose to be good to people right now?

TRAINING LOG: _____ miles or km _____ other training

Preparation Day 30:

Good character is not formed in a week or a month. It is created little by little, day by day. Protracted and patient effort is needed to develop good character. -Heraclitus

It's been a month but we're far from done. What things do you need to remind yourself to continue doing day by day?

TRAINING LOG: _____ miles or km _____ other training

Preparation Day 31:

"*Now, I hobble. OK? I trip all the time. I cannot use my right leg. My right arm and my right fingers do not work. I cannot type. I cannot manipulate things ... am I still an athlete? I say I am.*" – Jason Potsander

What's something you can't do anymore or don't do because it's too risky? How are you still the same person in spite of having given up that thing?

TRAINING LOG: _____ miles or km _____ other training

Preparation Day 32:

After climbing a great hill, one only finds that there are many more hills to climb. -Nelson Mandela

Today, go climb the biggest hill in the area. Look around, both outside yourself and inside, too. Where is the next metaphorical hill you must climb?

TRAINING LOG: _____ miles or km _____ other training

Preparation Day 33:
Now that you're in a rhythm with journaling, we'll leave more days blank, without prompts or without quotes, so you can write about whatever you want.

TRAINING LOG: _____ miles or km _____ other training

Preparation Day 34:
Great minds discuss ideas; average minds discuss events; small minds discuss people. -Eleanor Roosevelt
What's your big idea today?
TRAINING LOG: _____ miles or km _____ other training

Preparation Day 35: REST DAY

Think about one of your core values and brainstorm twenty ways to pass it on.

TRAINING LOG: _____ total miles completed in the last week.

Preparation Day 36:

You will never do anything in this world without courage. It is the greatest quality of the mind next to honor. -Aristotle

What requires courage as you train today or this week?

TRAINING LOG: _____ miles or km _____ other training

Preparation Day 37:
Notice the colors outdoors today. What did you see?
TRAINING LOG: _____ miles or km _____ other training

Preparation Day 38:
Push yourself a few extra minutes today. Not so much that it hurts, but just enough to say 'I did a little more than required.'
How do you feel about exceeding expectations?
TRAINING LOG: _____ miles or km _____ other training

Preparation Day 39:
Smell the air today. What does it smell like? Cows? Money? Disaster?
Write a poem about your favorite or least favorite smells.
TRAINING LOG: _____ miles or km _____ other training

Preparation Day 40:
The most wasted of all days is one without laughter. -e. e. cummings
Find something to laugh at today. A dumb joke. A ridiculous business idea. An improbable cause to support. What is the value of the absurd?
TRAINING LOG: _____ miles or km _____ other training

Preparation Day 41:
"All roads lead to Rome."
Where do all your roads lead? Where are you always going, even if you're coming home?
TRAINING LOG: _____ miles or km _____ other training

Preparation Day 42: REST DAY

As you approach the midway point of 90 days of training, it's time to increase the length of your longest walks. Plan something within the next week that adds at least a mile or two to your previous longest hike. For today, relax and recover.

TRAINING LOG: _____ total miles completed in the last week.

Preparation Day 43:
"A Stoic is someone who transforms fear into prudence, pain into transformation, mistakes into initiation, and desire into undertaking." — Nassim Nicholas Taleb
TRAINING LOG: _____ miles or km _____ other training

Preparation Day 44:
An examined life is a life worth living. -Peter Jansen
What have you been noticing about yourself this week?
TRAINING LOG: _____ miles or km _____ other training

Preparation Day 45:
Believe you can and you're halfway there. -Theodore Roosevelt
Halfway through 90 days of Camino training, your first 12 mile (21 km) day is coming up this week. What is the most challenging part of stretching to a longer distance? What concerns or fears do you have? What excites you about the challenge? What beliefs do you have now about your ability to do this?

TRAINING LOG: _____ miles or km _____ other training

Preparation Day 46:
Luck is a matter of preparation meeting opportunity. -Seneca
TRAINING LOG: _____ miles or km _____ other training

There's no shortcut to preparing to walk a Camino. It's time for a reality check. By the end of this week, you should have logged at least 195 miles (312 km) since day 1. If you got started late, put in extra miles here and there to catch up. Rate yourself based on what percentage you've achieved: 195 miles or more, full 100% – Doing great preparation.

175-194, 90% or better – Preparation is all right, but you'll need to step up over the next 6 weeks if you want to be lucky.

156-174 miles, 80% or better – You're behind. You're asking for some sore feet and sore muscles if you don't commit to the work now. If you continue at this pace, you'll probably still make it but it won't be fun.

136 to 155 miles, 70% or better. This isn't great. If you're in the higher end of this range you may be okay but if lower we'd have a concern that you'll have to abandon the Camino.

120 to 135. You can still take a shot at it but you need to add a mile to every one of your base workouts now. You're on the bubble. Ramp it up this week.

If you've logged 119 miles or fewer by now, it might be best to consider taking this trip later.

Preparation Day 47:
Take time to consider your mindset today. What do you need to tell yourself? What mental shifts are required?
TRAINING LOG: _____ miles or km _____ other training

Preparation Day 48:

I have met plenty of people who started a Camino without preparation, and it can be done, although you will suffer a lot more. But the physical preparation of walking many miles also prepares the mind to detach from the worries at home. If you're not doing that, you're going to miss the first half of your Camino– mentally– even while your body is on fire with pain, because you won't be ready to slow down enough to appreciate it.

How can you notice the slowing down beginning as you walk today?

TRAINING LOG: _____ miles or km _____ other training

Preparation Day 49: REST DAY

Today, instead of walking, try to sit and get to the same place in your head as you do when walking. You may call this meditation and do some breathing, or call it prayer and give your worries to the Creator, or simply think of it as 'stationary walking' and let your mind do the wandering. The point is to learn to slow down. Even if you're not used to meditating, you may find that because of the walking you've been doing, sitting still for 30 minutes won't be so difficult.

What did you observe?

TRAINING LOG: _____ total miles logged this week

Preparation Day 50:
Confidence comes from discipline and training. -Robert Kiyosaki
Name three things that you're more confident about now because of the training you've been doing.
TRAINING LOG: _____ miles or km _____ other training

Preparation Day 51:
Trusting our intuition often saves us from disaster. -Anne Wilson Schaef
As you walk today, think about what your intuition has been telling you lately. What disaster might be avoided by trusting your gut?
TRAINING LOG: _____ miles or km _____ other training

Preparation Day 52:

We are twice armed if we fight with faith. -Plato

What do you have faith for in yourself? What do you have faith for outside yourself?

TRAINING LOG: _____ miles or km _____ other training

Preparation Day 53:

"Victor said, 'You know, sometimes the mountain is on the inside.' And I said, 'Oh, I've climbed that mountain.'" -Susie Young-Tatum

What mountain inside yourself have you climbed before? Which one are you climbing today?

TRAINING LOG: _____ miles or km _____ other training

Preparation Day 54:

Do not attach yourself to materialistic things. Do not be a pawn in someone else's dream. - Miyamoto Musashi

As you walk today, consider what materialistic things you can detach from. How will this help you not be a pawn– or become the king or queen of your own dreams?

TRAINING LOG: _____ miles or km _____ other training

Preparation Day 55:
"Saint James walked there. He never walked back!" -Peter Jansen
Where are you going now that might be a place of no return? (This is your true mission.)
TRAINING LOG: _____ miles or km _____ other training

Preparation Day 56: REST DAY

Today is a day to sit still. Go out in nature (without taking too much of a hike) and sit still there. If it's raining, take a raincoat! Listen to the voice of the wild: What is it telling you today?

TRAINING LOG: _____ miles completed in the last week

Preparation Day 57:

I have never been lost, but I will admit to being confused for several weeks. -Daniel Boone

Take a different route today. If you're used to being in the city, go to the country. If you're used to walking in the country, hike through town. Think about being lost– what would it really mean to you to be lost?

TRAINING LOG: _____ miles or km _____ other training

Preparation Day 58:

Why does everyone think the future is space helmets, silver foil, and talking like computers, like a bad episode of Star Trek? -Tracey Ullman

In what ways does the natural world factor into your vision of the future?

TRAINING LOG: _____ miles or km _____ other training

Preparation Day 59:

I would feel more optimistic about a bright future for man if he spent less time proving that he can outwit Nature and more time tasting her sweetness and respecting her seniority. -E. B. White

As you walk outdoors today consider the sweetness and seniority of nature. Find a tree that has lived longer than you have. What is the best way to respect your elders today?

TRAINING LOG: _____ miles or km _____ other training

Preparation Day 60:
We're building up to some much longer walks. How do you feel about the Camino now that you've walked 12 miles in one day a few times?
TRAINING LOG: _____ miles or km _____ other training

Preparation Day 61:

A good traveler has no fixed plans and is not intent upon arriving." - Lao Tzu

As you plan for a longer walk in the next week, make time and create a route that will allow you to wander past a coffee shop, restaurant, and some other favorite places to sit and think. Feel free to take a break from your training during that walk and don't be so intent on arriving home. Don't treat every workout like a box to tick– soon you'll be on Camino and there won't be anything to do but travel.

TRAINING LOG: _____ miles or km _____ other training

Preparation Day 62:

"I was glib at best and probably dismissive at worst about this: The work of making this world resemble one that you would prefer to live in is a lunchpail f*cking job, day in and day out, where thousands of committed, anonymous, smart and dedicated people bang on closed doors and pick up those that are fallen and grind away on issues, 'til they get a positive result and even then, have to stay on to make sure that result holds. The good news is, I'm not saying you have to worry about who wins the election. I'm saying, you have to worry about every day before it, and every day after. Forever. Although, on the plus side, I am told at some point the sun will run out of hydrogen."

- Jon Stewart

As you walk today think about what closed doors are you banging on? What fallen people are you picking up? What issues are you grinding on? How are you taking these things one day at a time?

TRAINING LOG: _____ miles or km _____ other training

Preparation Day 63: REST DAY

Oh! do not attack me with your watch. A watch is always too fast or too slow. I cannot be dictated to by a watch. -Jane Austen

Enjoy resting today. How does it benefit you when you refuse to allow a watch to dictate your life?

TRAINING LOG: _____ mileage this week

Preparation Day 64:

"Time is a created thing. To say 'I don't have time,' is like saying, 'I don't want to.'" -Lao Tzu

What do you want to have time for? As we ramp up to our final training weeks, you'll need to ask yourself if you really want to commit the time to do the training. The ten, twelve, and even fifteen mile days. Decide that you want to, and again think about what you'll need to sacrifice to be able to finish this preparation.

TRAINING LOG: _____ miles or km _____ other training

Preparation Day 65:

"Greater love has no one than this: to lay down one's life for one's friends." -Jesus Christ

Think about this today: what friends would you give up your wealth for? What friends would you quit your job for? Who would you sacrifice everything you have to save? Who would you literally throw your body in front of a bullet for? Write down some of the people you care about most.

TRAINING LOG: _____ miles or km _____ other training

Preparation Day 66:
My doctor told me I would never walk again. My mother told me I would.
I believed my mother. -Wilma Rudolph
Who do you believe when it comes to what you could or could not do?
Who are the voices allowed to speak into that belief?
What do you appreciate about being able to walk?
TRAINING LOG: _____ miles or km _____ other training

Preparation Day 67:
A drawing is simply a line going for a walk. -Paul Klee
Think of yourself as a line today, and as you walk, think about what kind of drawing you are becoming.
TRAINING LOG: _____ miles or km _____ other training

Preparation Day 68:

People sacrifice the present for the future. But life is available only in the present. That is why we should walk in such a way that every step can bring us to the here and the now. -Thich Nhat Hanh

What do you take from today for today? How will that also be useful in the present when the future arrives?

TRAINING LOG: _____ miles or km _____ other training

Preparation Day 69:

Listen, real poetry doesn't say anything; it just ticks off the possibilities. Opens all doors. You can walk through any one that suits you. -Jim Morrison

What possibilities are opened today by the poetry of walking?

TRAINING LOG: _____ miles or km _____ other training

Preparation Day 70: REST DAY
The best way to predict the future is to create it. -Peter Drucker
   As you rest today reflect on how you have been predicting (creating) the
future throughout the last ten weeks.
   TRAINING LOG: _____ total miles over the last week.

Preparation Day 71:

This week you'll have your longest training day: 15 miles. Consider doing as much as 18 miles or six hours, if your body is in good form: if your feet are tough and you're not dealing with any injuries with sharp pains. Yes, your muscles will be sore, and your body will be tired.

How does it feel to know that you're nearly ready to go on your Camino?

TRAINING LOG: _____ miles or km _____ other training

Preparation Day 72:

If I lose forcing the pace all the way, well, at least I can live with myself. But if it's a slow pace, and I get beaten by a kicker who leaches off the front, then I'll always wonder, 'What if...?' -Steve Prefontaine

In general we are not training for a race, and we are working toward slowing down, and yet, there is an aspect of pushing the pace that we need for ourselves to rise to our best. This question isn't about how fast you walk, but how you can live with yourself. Where do you need to push the pace-or slow it down so that you can live with yourself? In your work, family or exercise routines? Somewhere else?

TRAINING LOG: _____ miles or km _____ other training

Preparation Day 73:
You get a lot of speeding tickets, and you say, 'I'm so unlucky!' No, you're not. You're speeding. Slow down. -D. B. Sweeney
Where is going too fast hurting you?
TRAINING LOG: _____ miles or km _____ other training

Preparation Day 74:

The longest journey is the journey inwards. Of him who has chosen his destiny, Who has started upon his quest for the source of his being. -Dag Hammarskjold

When did you start your quest for the source of your being? How does the journey inwards compare today with when you began?

TRAINING LOG: _____ miles or km _____ other training

Preparation Day 75:

I have great respect for the past. If you don't know where you've come from, you don't know where you're going. I have respect for the past, but I'm a person of the moment. I'm here, and I do my best to be completely centered at the place I'm at, then I go forward to the next place. -Maya Angelou

What is in your past that you pay respect to today while being in the moment?

TRAINING LOG: _____ miles or km _____ other training

Preparation Day 76:
Very little is needed to make a happy life; it is all within yourself, in your way of thinking. -Marcus Aurelius
What do you need to adjust in your way of thinking today?
TRAINING LOG: _____ miles or km _____ other training

Preparation Day 77: REST DAY

If you want to relax, watch the clouds pass by if you're laying on the grass, or sit in front of the creek; just doing nothing and having those still moments is what really rejuvenates the body. -Miranda Kerr

Sky, water, earth and fire: have a still moment with one of the four ancient elements today. Gaze into a campfire, watch a brook, investigate the nothing of the sky, or go to the beach to dig a hole in the sand with your hands. The Camino is coming up soon. What else can you do (or not do) to slow down today?

TRAINING LOG: _____ weekly miles total

Preparation Day 78:

Grit is living life like it's a marathon, not a sprint. -Angela Duckworth

On the Camino, you'll average a half-marathon every day– or more. This is your final week of training and you'll want to do two half-marathons (13.1 miles x 2) on back-to-back days. This means you'll walk a full Marathon in 48 hours. You should be doing it with a pack, too. So make sure to plan, it's a lot of walking.

What is it about the word Marathon, arbitrary as it may seem (26.2 miles) that you like or don't like? Does it intimidate or inspire and excite you? What other feelings come up when you hear the word "Marathon"? What does it mean to you to have grit?

TRAINING LOG: _____ miles or km _____ other training

Preparation Day 79:

When you run the marathon, you run against the distance, not against the other runners and not against the time. -Haile Gebrselassie

What has prepared you the most to go the distance: both the journey within and the long days of the Camino?

TRAINING LOG: _____ miles or km _____ other training

Preparation Day 80:
We have lost contact with reality, the simplicity of life. -Paulo Coelho
What is one simple reality you can reconnect with today, and how will you do it?
TRAINING LOG: _____ miles or km _____ other training

Preparation Day 81:

A life is not important except in the impact it has on other lives. -Jackie Robinson

In what ways are you impacting other lives?

TRAINING LOG: _____ miles or km _____ other training

Preparation Day 82:

Life isn't about finding yourself. Life is about creating yourself. -George Bernard Shaw

Who are you becoming as you create the new self today?

TRAINING LOG: _____ miles or km _____ other training

Preparation Day 83:
I dwell in possibility. -Emily Dickinson
Forever is composed of nows. -Emily Dickinson
Consider these two statements by Emily Dickinson. What is possible both now...
And now?
TRAINING LOG: _____ miles or km _____ other training

Preparation Day 84: REST DAY
Don't journal if you don't feel like it, today. If you do, start writing.
TRAINING LOG: _____ miles or km in the past week

Preparation Day 85:

Tapering off: the hardest part of training is done. If you've done well in terms of putting in the miles, you can consider taking an extra day off to allow your muscles, joints and ligaments to recover from the longest days.

Be honest with yourself: a few butterflies at the upcoming journey are normal. What is most satisfying about your preparation? What still concerns you?

TRAINING LOG: _____ miles or km _____ other training

Preparation Day 86:

Where would you be without friends? The people to pick you up when you need lifting? We come from homes far from perfect, so you end up almost parent and sibling to your friends - your own chosen family. There's nothing like a really loyal, dependable, good friend. Nothing. -Jennifer Aniston

It's time to think ahead to the Camino. You may walk alone quite a lot. Where has friendship helped you along the way? How will you extend it on the Camino, even when you're hot, cold, wet, rainy, tired, even exhausted? Make a commitment to yourself here:

TRAINING LOG: _____ miles or km _____ other training

Preparation Day 87:

The arts are not a way to make a living. They are a very human way of making life more bearable. Practicing an art, no matter how well or badly, is a way to make your soul grow, for heaven's sake. -Kurt Vonnegut

How have walking and journaling been an art form for you? How has your soul been growing as you write each day?

TRAINING LOG: _____ miles or km _____ other training

Preparation Day 88:

We never reflect how pleasant it is to ask for nothing. -Seneca

Try to make it through the day today while making as few requests as possible. What requests did circumstances require? How many times did people specifically ask you what you wanted? When you considered asking for something and opted not to, how did you feel?

TRAINING LOG: _____ miles or km _____ other training

Preparation Day 89:

The fear of death follows from the fear of life. A man who lives fully is prepared to die at any time. -Mark Twain

How have you lived fully? What fear, if any, do you have of death?

TRAINING LOG: _____ miles or km _____ other training

Preparation Day 90:
You're ready now. Enjoy your walk today. Think about this: When did your Camino really begin?
TRAINING LOG: _____ miles or km _____ other training

SECTION 3: TRAVEL DAYS

Travel Day 1: Use these days if traveling from home to a trail in another country or state will take you several days.

"Perhaps travel cannot prevent bigotry, but by demonstrating that all peoples cry, laugh, eat, worry, and die, it can introduce the idea that if we try and understand each other, we may even become friends." -Maya Angelou

Try striking up a conversation with someone, or if you're feeling bold, more than one person: in a taxi or Uber driver, in the airport, in the plane. Tell them you're doing research and ask them what was the last thing they laughed at. Journal: What do they have in common with you?

Travel Day 2:

"Why, I'd like nothing better than to achieve some bold adventure, worthy of our trip." -Aristophanes

The quote above suggests that a trip is one thing and an adventure is quite another. What do you think turns a trip into a "bold adventure"?

Travel Day 3:
There are no foreign lands. It is the traveler only who is foreign. -Robert Louis Stevenson
What kind of guest do you want to be?

SECTION 4: CAMINO WALKING DAYS

CAMINO WALKING DAY 1:

Welcome to the Camino, the next stage on your Legacy Way! What are your first impressions?

Today's Date:

Start:

End:

Miles/km hiked:

Who I walked with, met, or chatted with today:

CAMINO WALKING DAY 2:

"When the shoe fits, the foot is forgotten. When the belt fits, the belly is forgotten. When the heart is right, 'for' and 'against' are forgotten... Easy is right. Begin right and you are easy. Continue easy and you are right. The right way to go easy is to forget the right way and forget that the going is easy." -Chuang Tzu

What are you leaving behind, forgetting, today? Go easy, friends!

Today's Date:

Start:

End:

Miles/km hiked:

Who I walked with, met, or chatted with today:

CAMINO WALKING DAY 3:

"My brother is really, really slow." – Usain Bolt

Usually around the third day you'll begin to see that speed isn't relevant to the Camino. Try to find the stride that's just right for you and notice how your body feels when you walk this way: how do your feet, legs, torso, arms, neck and head feel? How does this impact your ability to go the distance?

Today's Date:

Start:

End:

Miles/km hiked:

Who I walked with, met, or chatted with today:

CAMINO WALKING DAY 4:

"It's your Camino. Walk it your way." – anonymous, ubiquitous saying on Camino de Santiago.

How are you beginning to make the Camino your own?

Today's Date:

Start:

End:

Miles/km hiked:

Who I walked with, met, or chatted with today:

CAMINO WALKING DAY 5:
"We have lost touch with reality, the simplicity of life." –Paulo Coelho
What are the simplest things you saw today? How do these things bring you in touch with reality?
Today's Date:
Start:
End:
Miles/km hiked:
Who I walked with, met, or chatted with today:

CAMINO WALKING DAY 6:

"The more I traveled the more I realized that fear makes strangers of people who should be friends." –Shirley Maclaine

Think about the people you've met so far. What is it about the openness of a Camino experience that helps you become friends so quickly?

Today's Date:

Start:

End:

Miles/km hiked:

Who I walked with, met, or chatted with today:

CAMINO WALKING DAY 7:

"Film is an illusion. Fame is ephemeral. Faith and family are what endure." – Emilio Estevez

Think about "walking into legacy" and how it compares to things that are not enduring. What has become truly important to you this week?

Today's Date:

Start:

End:

Miles/km hiked:

Who I walked with, met, or chatted with today:

CAMINO WALKING DAY 8:

"You're only here for a short visit. Don't hurry, don't worry. And be sure to smell the flowers along the way." – Walter Hagen

The Camino is really a short time in your life. What are some things you've done on this trip that help you learn not to hurry?

Today's Date:

Start:

End:

Miles/km hiked:

Who I walked with, met, or chatted with today:

CAMINO WALKING DAY 9:

"It took me four years to paint like Raphael, but a lifetime to paint like a child." – Pablo Picasso

What is your inner child discovering, drawing, and singing today? Today use your journal as a sketch pad. Draw little images from your time on the Camino.

Today's Date:

Start:

End:

Miles/km hiked:

Who I walked with, met, or chatted with today:

CAMINO WALKING DAY 10:

"Coincidence is God's way of remaining anonymous." – Albert Einstein

Think about people you've met and relationships you've built along the trail. Each one is a sort of coincidence: if you'd started two days earlier or later, you'd never have met. Which ones speak to you with a resounding message? How can you pay attention to that learning long-term?

Today's Date:

Start:

End:

Miles/km hiked:

Who I walked with, met, or chatted with today:

CAMINO WALKING DAY 11:

"If you cannot do great things, do small things in a great way." –
Napoleon Hill

What small things do you need to do daily to build toward your legacy,
even if they don't seem to be acts of greatness?

Today's Date:
Start:
End:
Miles/km hiked:
Who I walked with, met, or chatted with today:

CAMINO WALKING DAY 12:

"I like to take the formality out of the day's schedule and be ready for any off-road detour." – Matthew McConaughey

If you see a sign or an interesting note in a guidebook today, challenge yourself to go for a detour, fifty meters or five kilometers out of your way, practicing flexibility. What did you learn from the experience?

Today's Date:

Start:

End:

Miles/km hiked:

Who I walked with, met, or chatted with today:

CAMINO WALKING DAY 13:

"Walking with a friend in the dark is better than walking alone in the light." – Helen Keller

Today may be a good day to walk with a friend, even if only for an hour. Challenge yourself to listen. What's important to this other person? How does it relate to what's most important to you?

Today's Date:

Start:

End:

Miles/km hiked:

Who I walked with, met, or chatted with today:

CAMINO WALKING DAY 14:

"Everywhere is within walking distance if you have the time." – Steven Wright

Think about your legacy: you may not know how much time you have, but if you spend all your time moving toward it, what do you think could be within reach?

Today's Date:

Start:

End:

Miles/km hiked:

Who I walked with, met, or chatted with today:

CAMINO WALKING DAY 15:

"I understood at a very early age that in nature, I felt everything I should feel in church but never did. Walking in the woods, I felt in touch with the universe and with the spirit of the universe." – Alice Walker

Welcome to Alice Walker's cathedral. How do you feel in touch with God/spirit/universe today?

Today's Date:

Start:

End:

Miles/km hiked:

Who I walked with, met, or chatted with today:

CAMINO WALKING DAY 16:

"What fools call 'wasting time' is most often the best investment." –
Nassim Nicholas Taleb

What is the best investment you made today? What dividends can you anticipate?

Today's Date:

Start:

End:

Miles/km hiked:

Who I walked with, met, or chatted with today:

CAMINO WALKING DAY 17:

"I don't have to chase extraordinary moments to find happiness - it's right in front of me if I'm paying attention and practicing gratitude." – Brene Brown

Today may have an extraordinary moment, or it may not. What did you pay attention to today? What were you grateful for?

Today's Date:

Start:

End:

Miles/km hiked:

Who I walked with, met, or chatted with today:

CAMINO WALKING DAY 18:

"The true mystic is always both humble and compassionate, for she knows that she does not know." – Fr. Richard Rohr

Become aware today of the things you do not know. How does this humble you? How does it help you choose compassion?

Today's Date:

Start:

End:

Miles/km hiked:

Who I walked with, met, or chatted with today:

CAMINO WALKING DAY 19:
Go ahead. Write a poem today. Doesn't matter if it's good or not.
Today's Date:
Start:
End:
Miles/km hiked:
Who I walked with, met, or chatted with today:

CAMINO WALKING DAY 20:
"I asked myself about the present: how wide it was, how deep it was, how much was mine to keep." – Kurt Vonnegut
Today's Date:
Start:
End:
Miles/km hiked:
Who I walked with, met, or chatted with today:

CAMINO WALKING DAY 21:

"If a man does not keep pace with his companions, perhaps it is because he hears a different drummer. Let him step to the music which he hears, however measured or far away." – Henry David Thoreau

Where have you tried to keep pace with companions in life that has made it difficult to step within your own music? What might need to change when you return to daily life?

Today's Date:

Start:

End:

Miles/km hiked:

Who I walked with, met, or chatted with today:

CAMINO WALKING DAY 22:

"What makes the desert beautiful is that somewhere it hides a well." – Antoine de Saint-Exupery

Don't miss the beauty of finding a drink of water today, of finding shade, of finding the deep, hydrating draught of friendship. What is beautiful for you? What are the simplest things to be grateful for?

Today's Date:

Start:

End:

Miles/km hiked:

Who I walked with, met, or chatted with today:

CAMINO WALKING DAY 23:
At a certain point on Camino, it can be tempting to think that we are in such good condition that we are now become invincible, that there is no possibility of overdoing it.
What is enough for you today?
Today's Date:
Start:
End:
Miles/km hiked:
Who I walked with, met, or chatted with today:

CAMINO WALKING DAY 24:

"It is impossible to begin to learn that which one thinks one already knows." – Epictetus

Identify one assumption you have. What might you learn if you let go of that assumption?

Today's Date:

Start:

End:

Miles/km hiked:

Who I walked with, met, or chatted with today:

CAMINO WALKING DAY 25:
"Do not plan for ventures before finishing what's at hand." – Euripides
Some of our questions in this journal begin to hint at what will come next; be careful not to plan yet. Instead, write about your ideal future in a daydreaming sort of mode, or write a long list of options that you COULD do – but don't commit yet.
Today's Date:
Start:
End:
Miles/km hiked:
Who I walked with, met, or chatted with today:

CAMINO WALKING DAY 26:

"I never wanted to be the next Bruce Lee. I just wanted to be the first Jackie Chan." – Jackie Chan

When being the first you is at the height of awesomeness, what is happening?

Today's Date:

Start:

End:

Miles/km hiked:

Who I walked with, met, or chatted with today:

CAMINO WALKING DAY 27:

"Every autobiography is concerned with two characters, a Don Quixote, the Ego, and a Sancho Panza, the Self." – W. H. Auden

Even your journal is an autobiographical account of your journey. Which tends to emerge for you, the idealist, Quixote, or the realist, Sancho Panza?

Today's Date:

Start:

End:

Miles/km hiked:

Who I walked with, met, or chatted with today:

CAMINO WALKING DAY 28:

"When you arise in the morning, think of what a precious privilege it is to be alive - to breathe, to think, to enjoy, to love." – Marcus Aurelius

What do you consider a privilege today ... even if it hurts?

Today's Date:

Start:

End:

Miles/km hiked:

Who I walked with, met, or chatted with today:

CAMINO WALKING DAY 29:
"Every person has a legacy. You may not know what your impact is, and it may not be something that you can write on your tombstone, but every person has an impact on this world." – Dara Horn
Ah, but if you could write it on your tombstone, what would you like it to say?

Today's Date:
Start:
End:
Miles/km hiked:
Who I walked with, met, or chatted with today:

CAMINO WALKING DAY 30:

"The best remedy for those who are afraid, lonely, or unhappy is to go outside, somewhere where they can be quiet, alone with the heavens, nature, and God. Because only then does one feel that all is as it should be." – Anne Frank

Instead of journaling today, you may want to just sit under the heavens, in nature, with God. At the very least, ask for words to be given to you before you begin to write.

Today's Date:

Start:

End:

Miles/km hiked:

Who I walked with, met, or chatted with today:

CAMINO WALKING DAY 31:

"Aim for the sky, but move slowly, enjoying every step along the way. It is all those little steps that make the journey complete." – Chanda Kochhar

Think about all the small steps you've taken over 31 days of walking: it has been a full month of little steps. What have you enjoyed most about this month?

Today's Date:

Start:

End:

Miles/km hiked:

Who I walked with, met, or chatted with today:

CAMINO WALKING DAY 32:

"The voyage of discovery is not in seeking new landscapes but in having new eyes." – Marcel Proust

Think about the new eyes you have: what have you learned to see that was invisible to you before you began this journey?

Today's Date:

Start:

End:

Miles/km hiked:

Who I walked with, met, or chatted with today:

CAMINO WALKING DAY 33:

"Far better to be the simplest pedestrian, with knapsack on back, stick in hand, and gun on shoulder, than an Indian prince traveling with all the ceremonial which his rank requires." – Jules Verne

What is the best part about being 'the simplest pedestrian' today?

Today's Date:

Start:

End:

Miles/km hiked:

Who I walked with, met, or chatted with today:

CAMINO WALKING DAY 34:

"If an ass goes traveling he will not come home a horse." – Thomas Fuller

No doubt you have met some asses by now on your Camino. Let go of the fact that they are doing things in an asinine way. Give them permission to be who they are. Laugh it off before you reach your destination!

Today's Date:

Start:

End:

Miles/km hiked:

Who I walked with, met, or chatted with today:

CAMINO WALKING DAY 35:

"Some people are walking around with full use of their bodies and they're more paralyzed than I am." – Christopher Reeve

Your Camino draws to a close and it will soon be time to summon another kind of courage: what paralysis, what tranquilizer dart, must you remove so that you can walk into your purpose?

Today's Date:

Start:

End:

Miles/km hiked:

Who I walked with, met, or chatted with today:

CAMINO WALKING DAY 36:

"If you do not change direction, you may end up where you are heading."
– Lao Tzu

What have you chosen? What would you choose tomorrow if you feared no evil would come of it?

Today's Date:

Start:

End:

Miles/km hiked:

Who I walked with, met, or chatted with today:

CAMINO WALKING DAY 37:
"What I've found in my research is that realism and self-honesty are the antidote to ego, hubris, and delusion." – Ryan Holiday
Get real with yourself today.
Today's Date:
Start:
End:
Miles/km hiked:
Who I walked with, met, or chatted with today:

CAMINO WALKING DAY 38:

"If you reject the food, ignore the customs, fear the religion, and avoid the people, you might better stay at home." – James A. Michener

How have you embraced food, customs, people, and religious observances as you walked this Camino?

Today's Date:

Start:

End:

Miles/km hiked:

Who I walked with, met, or chatted with today:

CAMINO WALKING DAY 39:
"Life can only be understood backwards, but it must be lived forwards."
– Soren Kierkegaard
Your Camino draws to a close. What have you come to understand?
Today's Date:
Start:
End:
Miles/km hiked:
Who I walked with, met, or chatted with today:

CAMINO WALKING DAY 40 OR ARRIVAL AT FINAL HIKING DESTINATION

"Caminante, no hay camino, se hace camino al andar." (Walker, there is no way; you make a way by walking.) - Antonio Machado

You have walked for a long time now. You may feel relief, a letdown, elation ... Journal about your feelings, but also consider the question: what is the Way you have made?

Today's Date:

Start:

End:

Miles/km hiked:

Who I walked with, met, or chatted with today:

SECTION 5: CAMINO REST DAYS

CAMINO REST DAY 1:
Observe your surroundings. Enjoy. Eat. Take a nap. You are not getting behind. Some others may have gone on. You may see them again, or you may not. Rest in the ambiguity of it all. Rest today.

CAMINO REST DAY 2:

Go easy. Take it easy. There's nothing you have to do. If you see a museum, go ahead and wander around. The little bit of walking you do on a rest day can feel less like walking and more like wandering, and that's all right. Go to a grocery store or restaurant. Sit with friends and chat. Enjoy!

CAMINO REST DAY 3:

One of the great things about rest days on the Camino is that you don't have many chores to do. You can't paint the porch or wash the car. You may need to do some laundry, but really, what could be easier? Enjoy a good meal. Let your muscles rebuild.

CAMINO REST DAY 4:
Enjoy the company of old friends. Make some new ones. Invite someone for a coffee or tea, or beer or wine if you enjoy a drink now and then. These are the days to really learn to slow down; when you learn that to be on Camino does not even mean that you're always walking. Sometimes you walk, but sometimes you don't, and even that is okay.

CAMINO REST DAY 5:

Once in a while, we have a day where we do absolutely nothing. We make no progress. We pursue no goals. We restore our souls and bodies with sleep and food. Getting to a place where this is okay is paradoxically a step toward building our legacies.

CAMINO REST DAY 6:

Where would you be if you hadn't begun this sabbatical, this journey? How busy would you be today? Rest, friend, and be a friend to yourself as you rest. Accepting yourself as human means accepting that you must spend eight hours or so out of every twenty-four with your eyes closed. This is normal and healthy!

SECTION 6: RETURN TRAVEL DAYS

RETURN TRAVEL DAY 1:
"We shall not cease from exploration, and the end of all our exploring will be to arrive where we started and know the place for the first time." ~ T. S. Eliot
How do you plan to continue your exploration?
How might your return home allow you to really know it for the first time?

RETURN TRAVEL DAY 2:

"The power of finding beauty in the humblest things makes home happy and life lovely." ~ Louisa May Alcott

What beauty have you seen in humble things on Camino that you want to take home with you?

How will this help you make your home happy?

RETURN TRAVEL DAY 3:

"You can keep your willpower, Frog. I am going home to bake a cake." ~ Arnold Lobel

In one of Lobel's Frog and Toad books, Frog has been careful not to eat all the cookies, in deference to the principle of moderation. But moderation doesn't suit Toad.

What do you value at home that you can't enjoy while abroad? What are you looking forward to doing for pleasure now that you can relax a bit? In what ways do you need to maintain your disciplines? What core values do you want to ensure that you do not lose sight of, now that you are a Peregrino?

SECTION 7: DEBRIEF DAYS

DEBRIEF DAY 1:

Write down the ten memories from your Camino that you are most grateful for. They can be people you met or conversations, things you saw, tasted, or experienced...

DEBRIEF DAY 2:

Once a pilgrim, always a pilgrim: what do you hope will stay with you from the Camino for the rest of your life?

DEBRIEF DAY 3:
Reverse culture shock: what is it about daily life at home that now seems mundane, wasteful, or otherwise obnoxious? What can be done about this? How can you change or adapt to honor your Camino experience?

DEBRIEF DAY 4:

"Caminante, no hay camino, se hace camino al andar." (Walker, there is no path, the path is made by walking.) - Antonio Machado

Now that you've experienced what Machado meant, what is the path you have created?

DEBRIEF DAY 5:

Take a short walk today in a place where you commonly trained or prepared for your Camino. What do you notice about it now that you might not have noticed before?

DEBRIEF DAY 6:

As you begin to slip back into your routines at work and at home, don't wait too long to make the adjustments you planned. What needs to happen in the next week so that your new ideas can flourish?

DEBRIEF DAY 7:

"How does the true man of Tao [the way] walk through walls without obstruction, stand in fire without being burnt?

Not because of cunning or daring; not because he has learned, but because he has Unlearned." -Chuang Tzu

What have you unlearned and how does it allow you a certain invincibility?

DEBRIEF DAY 8:
Describe your most humbling experience on the Camino.

DEBRIEF DAY 9:
Describe the moment you came to the Cathedral (or other ending point).
How did it feel for the journey to be completed?
In what ways was your journey just beginning?

DEBRIEF DAY 10:
Think about a time when your body was exhausted but your spirit was soaring on the Camino.
How do you see the spirit, soul, and body linked together?

DEBRIEF DAY 11:
Sometimes people are concerned that taking so much time to go on Camino will be detrimental to their business, work or family. In what was are you beginning to see the benefits of this time away for your work or family?
How does it help put your legacy in focus?

Write about a friend you met on Camino. How did they impact or influence you?

DEBRIEF DAY 13:

Think about an interaction you had with someone local on the Way: an old lady selling fruit, a shop owner serving coffee and something to eat, a street performer, a museum curator... how did interacting with them (even if not speaking in the same language) influence your perspective on humanity?

DEBRIEF DAY 14:

Think about a time when you helped others on the Camino: Gave them ibuprofen, bought them lunch, shared an encouraging word or a hug or taught them a little trick you learned. Try to think of the smallest thing, something that cost you very little: how did it feel to offer someone your support in that moment?

Think about people you experienced as leaders on the Camino. Your coach or coaches, if you were on a Legacy Way Camino, or someone who gathered people into groups for a meal if on your own. How did it feel to be a part of that group, even if it was only one meal?

DEBRIEF DAY 16:
Think about people who were rude or at least indifferent to you during your Camino: bad drivers, shop owners who treated you poorly. Today, you can write a note of forgiveness to them. It is not worth allowing them to taint your experience.

DEBRIEF DAY 17:
Think about a time when you were impatient or rude on the Camino and didn't treat someone well. Today you can write a note of apology and also forgive yourself.

DEBRIEF DAY 18:

Some people (like the authors) find that a Camino experience is something to do more than once in a lifetime. If you don't think you'll ever do it again, that's totally fine.

How would you want your next experience to be different? In what ways would you like it to be the same?

DEBRIEF DAY 19:
Think about a time on the Camino when you really slowed down, and you found yourself truly in the moment. What was valuable about that for you?

DEBRIEF DAY 20:
How did the people you met on the Way influence the way you want to do relationships in the future: with colleagues, family, etc.?

DEBRIEF DAY 21:
How did the Camino reveal more about your innate nature to you? How was your understanding of self solidified?

DEBRIEF DAY 22:
How has the Camino made you more adaptable? Some components might be Grit, Mental Flexibility, Mindset, Resilience, and Unlearning.

DEBRIEF DAY 23:
Tomorrow, we'll start mapping out your Legacy Goal. Read the components on the next page and make some initial notes to yourself.
LEGACY goal components:

Lifetime and beyond: What are you working on now (or what do you want to begin today) that you hope will make the world a better place for your descendants or next-gen leaders?

Excellence: What aspects of the work require excellence? Do you need quality materials? Better craftsmanship? Or even improved marketing so that the work can be exploited properly for yield? What bad habits need to be eliminated to allow you to function with this excellence?

Generativity: What is it about your work that is generative? How is it creative and innovative, and what might be the next iteration or generation of the thing? What is the unique gift you are generating?

Audience: Who is it for? Who does your legacy serve? Is it your children, your customers, those who benefit from your nonprofit's services, or even your own employees?

Core Values Driven: As we mentioned in the section on Lifetime and Beyond, what core values might be the legacy itself? Besides Excellence in the areas you've already noted, what other core values must be in play at all times? Review your top five core values again: which ones are personal core values that others might not need to carry to be able to lead the next generation, and which ones are critical to the continuation of your legacy?

Yield: How does or will the legacy project also meet your needs?

$Yield^2$: What is your exit strategy? How will you be proactive so that Yielding is more of a *generous grant* than a reluctant surrender?

DEBRIEF DAY 24: LEGACY

LIFETIME and BEYOND: What are the things you're working on that you hope will outlive you?

DEBRIEF DAY 25: LEGACY

EXCELLENCE: In what areas do you need to increase your excellence so that you'll be able to pass on your LEGACY?

DEBRIEF DAY 26: LEGACY

GENERATIVE: What are you birthing into the world that is unique and beautiful? What are you making, creating, innovating, or tweaking?

DEBRIEF DAY 27: LEGACY
AUDIENCE: Even if it's only one person, who is your LEGACY for? Who are you serving? Who will benefit from what you've built?

DEBRIEF DAY 28: LEGACY
CORE VALUES DRIVEN: List your top ten Core Values. Then identify your top three to five. Bonus question: what image illustrates that core value for you? (Example: I use an oak tree to symbolize strength, I use a falcon to symbolize speed...)
NOTE: You can also use the core values exercise at the back of the journal.

DEBRIEF DAY 29: LEGACY

YIELD (first definition): How does your LEGACY include a return on investment that also sustains you? What is the crop or harvest or profit? How are you using that today to not only take care of your own needs but reinvest in the LEGACY?

DEBRIEF DAY 30: LEGACY

YIELD (second definition): What is your exit strategy? How will you pass on what you've built, learned, been given, designed, created and cared for? How will you pass on the core values that got you where you are today?

How are you training leadership in your legacy? How open is your communication about your exit strategy?

Things to do if you haven't already done them: Make a will. Talk with your children, your board, or with your "heirs to the throne" about your wishes.

I developed the list of 40 words below by combining core values lists from several different sources, until I had a list of more than 500 words. Many of those words overlapped, and I felt the list was overwhelming, so I began to categorize them. For example, I grouped these 12 words:

Accomplishment, Advancement, Ambition, Capability, Drive, Growth, Impact, Improvement, Make a Difference, Pursuit, Significance, and Success.

Next, I titled the group "Achievement." All 40 words in the master list below were headings for groups of five to fifteen other words from my original list of 500+. The list is intended as a thinking prompt. It's okay if you don't end up with any of them in your top five. There is no perfect list.

How to: Circle the five that resonate the most, or write down words you already know are in your top core values. Then use a thesaurus to expand your search for words that fit you even better. Do this even for words you've considered your top core values for years with an open mind and see if you can sharpen your list. For example, my top core value is Friendship, but it's not on this list. You can imagine that I might come to Friendship through thinking about Acceptance, Fun, Love, or Stability.

Acceptance	Education	Honor	Responsibility
Achievement	Excellence	Hospitality	Risk-taking
Awareness	Flexibility	Humility	Spirituality
Beauty	Focus	Justice	Stability
Competition	Freedom	Love	Strength
Connection	Fun	Order	Sustainability
Creativity	Generosity	Passion	Thankfulness
Curiosity	Hard-working	Peace	Uniqueness
Diversity	Health	Prosperity	Vision
Economy	Honesty	Reputation	Wisdom